How to Sleep Like a Bear
Putting Insomnia to Bed

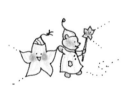
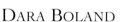

Dara Boland

CELESTIAL ARTS

Berkeley • Toronto

Note to the Reader
This book is not intended to be a substitute for professional medical care or the advice of a physician. We recommend that you seek the guidance of a licensed health care provider before following the advice in this book.

Celestial Arts
P.O. Box 7123
Berkeley, California 94707
www.tenspeed.com
A Heart & Star book

Distributed in Canada by Ten Speed Press Canada, in the United Kingdom and Europe by Airlift Books, in New Zealand by Southern Publishers Group, in Australia by Simon & Schuster Australia, in South Africa by Real Books, and in Singapore, Malaysia, Hong Kong, and Thailand by Berkeley Books.

Illustrations by Dara Boland
Book and cover design by Larissa Pickens

Grateful acknowledgment is made to the publishers for the use of the following copyrighted material: Text on page 3 from *Traditional Chinese Medicine* by Sheila McNamara. Copyright © 1995 by Sheila McNamara and Dr. Song Xuan Ke. Reprinted by permission of Basic Books, a member of Perseus Books, L.L.C.

Quote on page 77 from *Spirits of the Earth* by Bobby Lake-Thom, copyright © 1997 by Bobby Lake-Thom. Used by permission of Plume, a division of Penguin Putnam Inc.

Text on page 30 reprinted with permission of Simon & Schuster from *Earthway: A Native American Visionary's Path to Total Mind, Body and Spirit Health* by Mary Summer Rain. Copyright © 1990 by Mary Summer Rain.

Text on page 94 reprinted with permission of John Wiley & Sons, Inc. from *No More Sleepless Nights* by Peter Hauri, Ph.D. and Shirley Linde, Ph.D. New York: John Wiley and Sons, Inc., copyright © 1990.

Library of Congress Cataloging-in-Publication Data
Boland, Dara.

How to sleep like a bear: putting insomnia to bed / Dara Boland.

p. cm.
Includes bibliographical references.
ISBN 0-89087-975-3
    1. Insomnia—Popular works.   I. Title.
    RC548.B64 2000
    616.8′498—dc21

2001001600

First printing, 2001
Printed in Hong Kong

1 2 3 4 5 6 7—05 04 03 02 01

Dedication

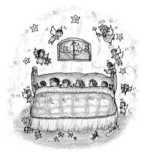

For
Michael, Matthew, and Kathryn Boland
Mollie, Abby, and Emily Thompson
&
Woody
and
Rebecca

May you always be watched
over by angels,
asleep or awake.

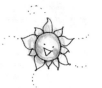

Acknowledgments

The angels that watch over us as we sleep speak to us through souls here on earth, helping us believe in what we were sent here to do in the first place. Mine are as follows:

First and foremost, Alice Martell. You believed in me from the beginning. You *are* my beginning in the work I always dreamed of doing.

Kathryn Ettinger, my editor and friend, I thank you from the bottom of my heart for turning my hodgepodge project into the message I meant to convey to everyone who wants the peace of good sleep. I thank you, Celestial Arts, for another opportunity to do what I so love to do.

Annie Nelson, I am so grateful to you for expertly picking up where Kathryn left off, and to Shirley Coe and Larissa Pickens for your expertise.

Thanks to Danielle Turner and Jean Gordner for your help; to Ann Jones of Herb Works and the folks at Just Desserts Bakery, both in Cary, North Carolina, for all your sleepy suggestions; Patricia Schmidt for the information on Watsu; thanks to Janice Mancuso, author of *Herbed Wine Cuisine* and friend; and thanks to David Bonomo for yawning and walking away when I said, "I can't."

Many thanks to Sue and Bill Wittman, Aunt Lynn and Uncle Tom Cianflone, and Lynn and Mark Thompson; Stephanie Lovett; Julie Jallád; Vicki Denison and Jackie Bonomo; and Joyce, Mark, and Krista Boland, who helped me to believe in myself.

Thanks to Nannie, who warmed up my socks on the heater so I didn't have to get out of bed with a chill when I was so sick, and to Boppie, my inspiration. And of course, thank you to my parents, Kevin and Jean Boland, for tucking me in every night for all those years, no matter what.

You have all helped make my sweetest dreams come true.

Table of Contents

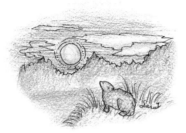

*"Come forth into the light of things,
Let nature be your teacher."*

~ William Wordsworth

I. INTRODUCTION

ou've been to the doctor.
You've rearranged the bedroom.
You bought a $50 pillow.
You've tried eye patches, ear plugs,
sound machines, and subliminal tapes.
You've been to a shrink.
And still
you just can't sleep.
Or falling asleep is no problem, but staying there *is*.

When you have insomnia, you *know* you can't sleep.
You may even have a good idea *why*.
So the task lies not in looking at the sleep itself
(which we cannot do), but in looking around the sleep
at all those other things we do too much:

• dwelling on thoughts while we're lying there, staring at moonlit walls

• yearning for what we don't have during the day

• feeling overwhelmed by the stresses of the past, present, and future
and how we handle (or fail to handle) them

No pill can cure these things.

Insomnia Is a Teacher

lthough it may not seem so when it's 3 a.m. and you're
lying there thinking of your 6 a.m. wake-up call,
your seeming inability to get a good night's rest
is the wake-up call.
Something in your *waking life* needs fixing, and
only you can do the fixing. But what you believe is
broken may or may not be what really needs repair.
You need to go back to the
real source ~ and look inside your heart.

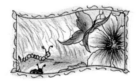

At
this point
in your life,
what do *you* think
needs fixing?

What do you *believe* your insomnia is trying to teach you?

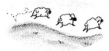

In traditional Chinese medicine, the heart is the home of one's spirit or "heart fire." Ideally, one's spirit lives in the mind by day and goes home to the heart by night. *Qi*, the vital energy that moves through your body via the blood, flows unblocked. The kidneys, ruled by water, "put out" excess heart fire so that it does not overrun everything else within us. Thus, a natural system of checks and balances keeps our mind-body functioning harmoniously.

But what happens when the natural flow of *Qi* is interrupted and the balance is thrown off? Insomnia, among other things.

Insomnia is treated in Eastern medicine as a displaced spirit ~ at the very least, a distracted one. When the blood is diverted to an overstressed area of the body ~ the uterus in the case of PMS-related insomnia, for example ~ instead of returning home to the heart at night, the result is "empty heart fire." This deficiency causes a restless, hungry spirit at night.

This makes perfect sense to those whose insomnia is related to some other condition ~ physical or psychological. If you suspect you are suffering from depression or if you have any other symptoms besides a seeming inability to sleep, you need a doctor's help. Curing the underlying illness is necessary before your insomnia can leave you.

But if your physician has ruled out illness, your sickness may be one of the very spirit that is looking for a place in your heart at night.

"Empty heart fire" is a sickness of the soul.

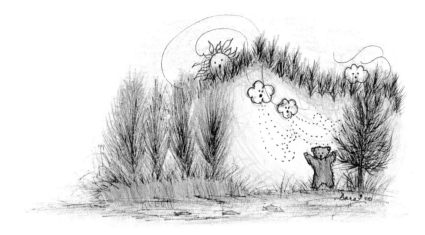

Like a flooded river that overflows,
a flooded mind cannot be contained and will keep you awake at night.
Your soul may be yearning for some kind of freedom, such as

a meaningful career
or
a more meaningful way of looking at the one you already have.

Or the idea for a novel may be roaming around in your
brain, the one you've always dreamed you'd write.
(If there is a story inside you, aching to break free, it *will*
keep you up at night. Trust me on that one!)

Let It Out and You Will Sleep

The challenge, of course,
is finding out what

"it"
is.

Unearth the *source*
of your insomnia. Like a bear
scratching through pine needles for bugs,
dig until you can find it.
Look at it, ingest it, and fully digest it
so you can get on with the real work of living and resting.
Then you can put insomnia to bed for good.
Insomnia is, after all, a pest!

II. How Bears Sleep

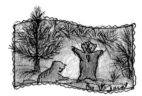

hi · ber · nate: to spend the winter in a dormant state

~ *Webster's New World Dictionary*

- Hibernation is more than a retreat. When the weather gets colder and the days get shorter, hibernation is necessary for bears, as food becomes scarce. Sleep is a survival mechanism; without this downtime a bear's energy needs could not be met.

- Not all bears hibernate the same way. Male Florida black bears and most male polar bears barely settle down for that long winter's nap. Mexican black bears "den up" for only a few short weeks, while black bears in the Yukon may hibernate for several months. Hibernation styles can vary even within individual bear populations.

- Female bears build a den in late fall, where they give birth to their cubs, usually in February. The cubs are around the size of squirrels when they are born, but by springtime they may weigh upwards of twenty pounds! (Not bad for a nursing mom with no food to eat, is it?)

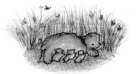

- Contrary to common belief, bears do wake up during hibernation. A mother bear, especially, will attack if she senses danger to her cubs. If there's no danger, the awakened bear will readjust her bedding, check on (or lick) the cubs, and doze off again. Male bears are very territorial and don't particularly care for intruders, either. Like many humans, bears are partial to staying asleep once they get there, and tend to be grouchy when awakened unexpectedly.

- The scent of spring air and longer hours of daylight rouse a bear from sleep. (Some alarm clock, right?) Males venture out first, then females. Mothers with cubs emerge last to a buffet of berries and plants that awaits them.

Hibernation is a time for rest, renewal, and rebirth for bears, just as sleep can be for us. While you work on your sleep issues, consider resting peacefully *physically* as a great accomplishment. Your nightly dormancy may consist of reading or listening to soft music in a reclining position. This may be all you can manage right now, and that's okay.

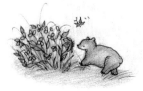

III. How to Sleep Like a Bear

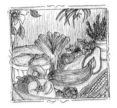

"The healer of disease is Nature."

~ Hippocrates

We humans can learn a lot about sound sleep from bears:

- Some bears hibernate longer than others. Some of us need more sleep in order to function at an optimum level. As we age, we may need less sleep. Then again, we could be needing *more* sleep, if we are still leading the same hectic lifestyle of our younger days.

- Bears make their own dens out of available materials *to their individual liking*. Creating your own comfortable sleeping space requires time, energy, and thought. Some of us need a more *tailored* space than others; everybody (bear, human, or otherwise) is unique.

Dens, like bedrooms, are havens of quiet, rest, and solitude. Bears use their dens just as we need to on a daily basis: to recharge our batteries so our waking hours can be fruitful.

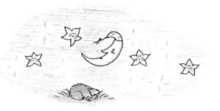

Why don't bears get insomnia and I do???!!!

- Bears, like all of nature's creatures (with the exception of humans), don't try to be superheroes. There's a lot about life that bears can't control, but, unlike us, they move on. A bear knows instinctively that nature moves in cycles. He trusts the natural flow of things and his ability to function within the parameters of an ever-changing world. Terrifying stuff to us humans.

- A bear doesn't hang around and lament an empty berry patch. He uses what energy he has from previous berries in order to find more food elsewhere.

And so it should be with us.

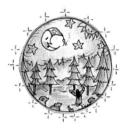

*"'I just had another dream,' Joseph said.
'The sun and moon and eleven stars were bowing down to me.'"*

~ Genesis 37:9

Why do you believe you are here? What and who do you love? Are you with that person or persons, putting yourself in settings where it all "clicks" for you? Are you clinging to a dying berry bush—an old way of doing things, a career, a hometown, or a relationship that just isn't working for you anymore? What gives your life meaning and purpose? Are you dreaming it, or are you living it?

Bears and all of nature's creatures operate on the *"No Dress Rehearsal"* rule. They live their lives with an authenticity many of us yearn for but few of us take the steps to achieve. They take care of business as they see fit, without worrying about expectations others may have of them.

When you have trouble sleeping, something may be amiss in how you are living your days, something that is keeping you from the renewal you deserve each night. Something that is, quite literally, keeping you from your dreams.

Exercise

I f you often lie awake at night with random thoughts racing through or lollygagging around in your mind, something about the truth of You may be trying to push through to your conscious mind. The following may help unearth that truth:

1. Picture yourself in the woods. Through a clearing in the trees an image takes shape ~ it is your Creator. This could be your mother and father, a deity, or a god-like being. It could be a bear or a goddess—whatever fits for you. Now ask this image the following:

    • *"Why was I put here on earth?"*

    Now imagine the answer. Keep in mind that this answer may have little to do with how you live your life now, or it may contain many elements of your current lifestyle.

    Creator's answer:

    _____

    _____

    _____

    _____

    _____

    _____

    _____

2. Okay, maybe that one was too weird for you. Try this one:

Once upon a time, _____ (your name here) was born. He/she dreamed of becoming a _____. He/she grew up in _____ (hometown) and moved to _____ (current home) and became a _____ (occupation). If he/she could have, he/she would have lived in _____ (name a place) and lived the lifestyle of a _____. He/she could still do these things if only:

_____

_____

He/she is waiting for:

_____

_____

3. Now put it in your own words. What I really live for is:

_____

_____

_____

The world wants what you have to give. *Really.*

Promise yourself that you will explore a new berry patch
(or whatever strikes your fancy) each and every day. And at night

do as the bears do and...

• fluff up your den so that it is comfortable to you

• be sure it is quiet and secluded

• don't go to bed hungry

• stay cool

• get up and walk around if you wake up

• patiently get comfortable again

~ and ~

let yourself doze off...

How Do You Sleep Like a Bear?

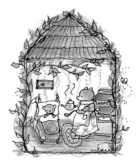

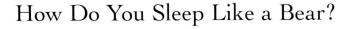ou come to learn ~ for the first time, perhaps ~ how to trust yourself enough to do what you need to do by day so your sleeping hours are for sleep and are not "Should have done" and "Can't forget to do" time. Bedtime can truly mean ~ *for you* ~ a time for rest and renewal, as it is for the rest of nature's children!

In order to sleep the natural way ~ the bear's way ~ you must learn to:

1. Surrender to Your Insomnia
2. Prepare Your Lair
3. Listen to Your Chattering Mind
4. Weather the Storm
5. Mother Yourself to Sleep

Why don't adults, like the children we once were, get nap time?

Getting comfortable again with sleep...
hmmmmmmmmm...

1. Surrender to Your Insomnia

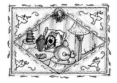

"The only thing we have to fear is fear itself."

~ Franklin D. Roosevelt,
First Inaugural Address, March 4, 1933

Insomnia ~ *The Vicious Circle*

When I had insomnia I dreaded going to bed. Pretty soon the mere *thought* of bedtime was enough to send me into a panic. Perhaps the same has happened with you: insomnia generates an anxiety about insomnia, which in turn just causes more insomnia.

The cycle goes like this:

1. You can't sleep.
2. You dread bedtime.
3. You can't sleep ~ again.
4. You worry you won't ever get a good night's rest.
5. You can't sleep again.
6. You worry about your impending crankiness and inability to face the following day at your best.
7. You can't sleep again, and so on.

I hate to bring up math at a time like this, but ...remember this?

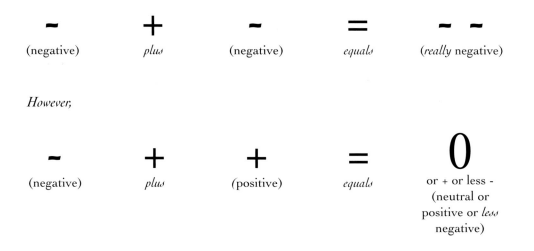

~ (negative)   *plus*   ~ (negative)   =   ~ ~ (*really* negative)

However,

~ (negative)   *plus*   + (positive)   =   0 or + or less - (neutral or positive or *less* negative)

Now let's apply this to insomnia. If insomnia were an equation, it would look like this:

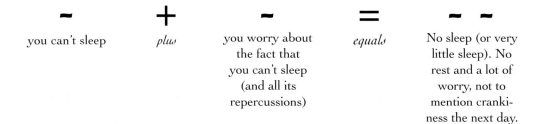

~ you can't sleep   *plus*   ~ you worry about the fact that you can't sleep (and all its repercussions)   =   ~ ~ No sleep (or very little sleep). No rest and a lot of worry, not to mention crankiness the next day.

So...
how do we get from insomnia to sleep?

Add a positive.

−	**+**	**+**	**=**	**0**
(negative)	*plus*	(positive)	*equals*	or + or less −
You can't sleep.		You picture yourself sleeping soundly in vivid detail, and you agree to give yourself some physical rest, if not sleep.		You can't sleep, but you rest your weary bones.

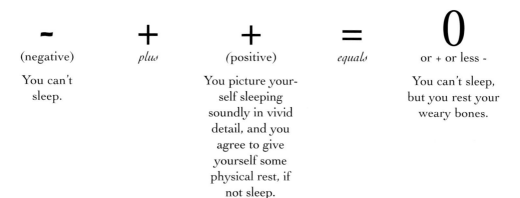

At first you may still worry about being able to sleep. Old habits die hard. But go ahead and add a positive anyway. It can't hurt, and it will probably help.

As far-fetched as this plan may sound to you, you are in a fragile state right now if you haven't been sleeping. And positive, mother bear-like comfort may salve your tired spirit. The hardest part is doing the *mental* work and remembering to add the positive.

If your body still won't sleep, let your mind help you relax. Even if you don't get a great night's rest, you can still break the cycle of worrying yourself into more insomnia.

The equation looks like this:

–	+	+	=	0
(negative)	*plus*	(positive)	*equals*	(somewhere closer to *neutral*)
You can't sleep *again.*		You get up and comfort yourself with a repetitive activity like needlepoint, rolling up pennies, even some light cleaning.		Eventually you get some sleep. It may be great or just okay, but it's much better than before.

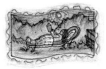

*"...will your worship with all your power
be able to make me sleep if I don't choose to?"*

~ Miguel de Cervantes,
The Adventures of Don Quixote

Homeopathy is based on the ancient wisdom that a small dose of what ails you will help your body come to its own defense. This is the principle behind immunizations; you may feel a bit sick after getting a flu shot because the shot actually contains the flu. By the time you are exposed to a flu bug, your body has built up antibodies to fight off the illness. The notion that "like cures like" can be applied to insomnia as well.

Face your insomnia.

Accept it, *surrender to it,* work with it. Like a mother bear who awakens from a deep winter sleep to defend her young, you must confront the source of your sleeplessness and, eventually, rise up to the challenge.

The reason for the disturbance will remain if you do not get up and deal with it. And how do you deal with not being able to sleep?

By not trying to sleep.

You will be more tired and *more* irritable tomorrow if you spend the night battling with yourself, attempting to force your mind to sleep. The *opposite* is called for: gentle kindness toward sleepless you.

Give Yourself a "Sleep Expectation Break"

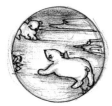

Many insomniacs are perfectionists, also known as "either-or thinkers": "*Either* I can sleep six or eight straight hours *or* I can't, and I'll be irritable and inept tomorrow."

Lower your expectations.

The thought of eight straight hours of sleep may be too high an expectation for you right now. The human body needs to sleep, to be sure. But resting peacefully is much more beneficial than tossing and turning and stressing yourself about being unable to sleep. Rather than thinking in black and white ("I must have a good night's sleep *now!*"), shoot for gray ("I'll just rest my body and that will be okay."). Instead of believing you *must* go to sleep and you *must* sleep straight through the night, unwind as much as possible (more on that later) and promise yourself that you will try to sleep for a couple of hours. Simply *take a nap*.

Sometimes just knowing you don't *have to* (we have enough have-tos during the day) sleep is enough to help you relax to the point of real sleep!

Performance anxiety cannot exist without the expectation for excellence!

Work with who you are *today*.

Accept the fact that,
just for now,
resting your body
is all you can do.

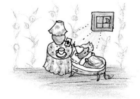

For now, that is
your form
of sleep.

And let it rest.

Underneath it all
you are one of nature's creatures
like bears and birds and flowering trees.

Many of the pressures and responsibilities of our modern world are not very natural at all. We were not built to sit in front of computer screens all day. We were not designed to sit in traffic and fret about money.

So what do you do?

You don't change your entire life.

You don't move away, because surely
the same old problems will eventually follow.

You do dig deep back to the natural part of you,
that so needs to trust that things will work out okay,
and that no matter what, there's only so much you control.

The rest is up to nature.

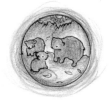

Insomnia: A Lesson in Letting Go

- *Respect* yourself (the nature within you).

- Respect the nature around you.

- Do what you *can*.

- Practice *letting go* of the rest.

Imagine yourself literally flinging
your leftover concerns into the air.
You may still feel them, but stand your ground.
Like a bear searching for salmon against a strong river
current, plant your feet in shallow
water and stay still.
Let your concerns be carried away with the current...

This may be the hardest thing you've ever done.
Many of us insomniacs have a terrible time letting go
and letting things happen naturally.
But just the act of practicing this
is
progress.

You may find a lot of room
waiting to be filled with self-kindness.

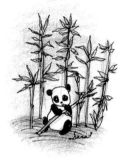

BEAR FACT

Unless it is storming
or she is giving birth,
a panda will sleep on
the ground, wherever she
happens to be, whenever she
feels tired enough to
rest.

2. Prepare Your Lair

"I've often told my decorating clients that they should love everything in their house."

~ Alexandra Stoddard,
Gracious Living in a New World

When bears get ready to hibernate, they choose a spot, usually not far from last year's location (if it worked well), that is far removed from noise, distraction, and danger.

Setting up camp involves digging through branches and twigs, or snow in the case of polar bears, then laying down some grasses, or packing down some snow, for suitably soft but firm bedding.

Any bear can tell you: the best spot to sleep is *both* found and made.

Look around your bedroom:
>Is this a place you'd *want* to sleep in?
>• Your "cozy" may be someone else's "claustrophobic."
>• What is streamlined to one may be clinical to another.
>• Comfortably cool to you can be freeeezing to someone else.

Visualize Your Ideal Den

Imagine your ideal sleeping space. What do you see? Is the room airy and bright, full of plants and adornments? Or are the lines clean and simple? Is it dark and cozy, full of overstuffed pillows, tapestries, and throws?

Now imagine yourself in that space, feeling relaxed and ready to go to sleep. Picture the look on your face as you settle into bed and turn out the lights.

Write what you see and feel:

My ideal sleep spot looks: _____ .

It makes me feel: _____ .

My bed is: _____ .

The room smells like: _____ .

I'm ready to go to sleep because: _____ .

If I could change three things about my current sleep spot by tonight I would:

1. _____

2. _____

3. _____

I promise to do the following as a gift to my tired self in an effort to make my current sleep space more like my ideal den:

1. _____

2. _____

3. _____

Don't lie there stewing about it.
Look *around* your insomnia!

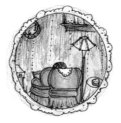

Look around you. What conditions contribute to or detract from your favorable sleep environment?

All of nature's beings, it seems, are affected by air quality and atmospheric conditions. Think about what's going on "out there" (outside your bedroom) and how it's affecting you "in here" (inside your body):

Outside Your Bedroom

- What is your favorite season?
- Do you sleep better when it's cold out?
- Or at the first signs of spring?
- Does a dry heat really make a difference to the quality of your sleep?
- Do the first signs and sounds of autumn send you into overdrive?
- Or are you a summer sleeper, happily drifting off with a light nocturnal breeze from an open window, waking to the scent of sun in the air? (Can't you just *smell* a pretty day?)

Inside Your Skin

- Pay attention to your body temperature tonight. If you go to bed or wake during the night feeling uncomfortably warm, try lowering the thermostat or sleeping in layers of nightwear, which can be peeled off if need be. If it's chilly, keep extra blankets at the bottom of your bed. If you wake up parched and thirsty at night, a humidifier and some leafy plants can restore moisture to your bedroom air, regardless of the season.

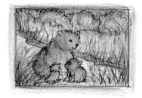

BEAR FACT

The winter weight a bear packs on prior to hibernation is the ultimate blanket.
It gets thinner and lighter as the weather warms up!

- Are you a beach person? If so, do you live near a body of water? Do you sleep more soundly when rain tickles your roof? The sight or sound of water may lull you to sleep; a fish tank, a tabletop fountain, or a CD of ocean sounds may soothe you.

- Are you a country person living in a city? Traffic noise, crowded stores and streets and roads, and houses and apartments too close together may be bugging you on a deeper level than you realize.

Think of a Time When You *Could* Sleep

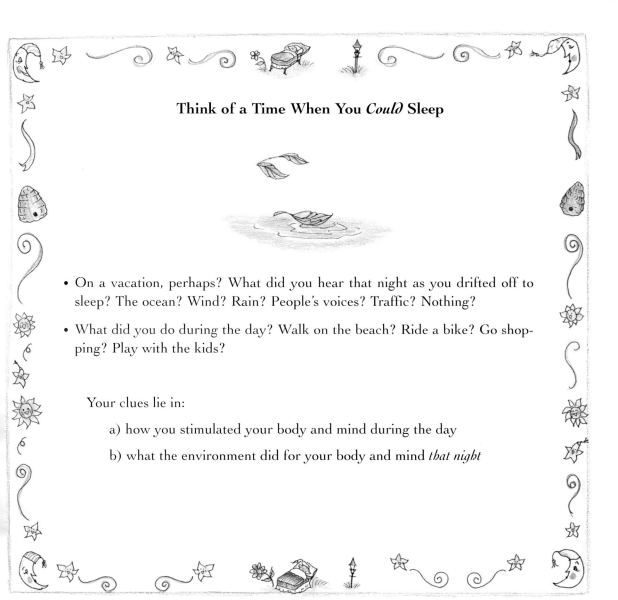

- On a vacation, perhaps? What did you hear that night as you drifted off to sleep? The ocean? Wind? Rain? People's voices? Traffic? Nothing?

- What did you do during the day? Walk on the beach? Ride a bike? Go shopping? Play with the kids?

Your clues lie in:

    a) how you stimulated your body and mind during the day

    b) what the environment did for your body and mind *that night*

Furniture Placement for Peace of Mind

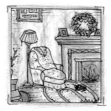

From feng shui to ergonomics, it has been known for centuries that the composition, shape, and placement of furniture either promotes flow and inner harmony or hinders them.

- Native American wisdom teaches that a north-facing headboard will reward you with a good sleep. This places you in alignment with the magnetic pull of the earth so all those busy thoughts that keep you awake at night can be drawn out.

- Natural materials (wood, clay, stone) are recommended for your bedroom decor as opposed to man-made metal items. Circular objects are said to promote unity, reflecting the circular nature of our world. The idea is to bridge the gap between your inner world and your external world.

- Let the placement of your belongings and the flavor of your surroundings be a reminder of the peace you want more of. It's bound to have a balancing effect on your psyche.

Hey, it's worth a try, right?

Nature Doesn't Speak in Words

Pay attention to your instincts. Your senses can provide important hints to help cure your insomnia.

Right at this moment...

What do you hear?
What kind of taste do you have in your mouth?
Look around you:
Is the scene around you peaceful?
      Chaotic?
How do you *feel* about what you see?
What does that feeling remind you of from your past?
Do you smell something?
Do you have a headache? Backache? Shoulder ache?

S - t - r - e - t - c - h gently.

How are you breathing?
Long, relaxed breaths or short, shallow ones?
(Many of us hold our breath under stress.)

Become aware of your surroundings and your internal response to them.

The clues you need for healing your insomnia
may be found in individual moments
and how you experience them.

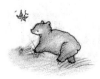

Use All Your Senses to Find Your "Cure"

1. Smell. Bears have a very keen sense of smell. Smelling something good (like delicious edible grasses) or sniffing something bad (like an intruder) greatly determines their actions. Although our sense of smell is not as fine-tuned as that of a bear, what we do and do not smell can influence our capacity for a sound sleep.

- Lavender oil has a soothing effect on the nerves and the nose. You can massage lavender-scented oil onto your wrists or your feet. (Note: Essential oils are potent and must be diluted with a vegetable oil "carrier" before being applied to your skin. Always read the label for instructions or consult a certified herbalist for proper dosages.) A lavender sachet beneath your pillow or a spritz of lavender spray in your bedroom can also help relax you.

- The smell of perfume or stale cigarette smoke on clothes hanging in your closet can aggravate your sense of smell.

- A stuffy bedroom might seem cozy at bedtime but can become stifling in the middle of the night. Hidden molds or mildews ~ in an adjoining bathroom, in window jambs, in and around the bottom of the house, or in heating and air vents and pipes ~ can aggravate sinuses and make breathing difficult. A few sniffles could mean a good cleaning is in order!

2. Sight. Your bedroom is your sanctuary for sleep. Treat your eyes to your version of visual peace.

- Look around your bedroom. Are you surrounded by comforting sights? Is this a room you want to sleep in? You should *love* everything in your room. Even simple touches ~ tie-backs on your curtains, throw pillows, whimsical decorations, dolls, or toys ~ can help you feel more at home. A potted plant can be a welcome addition to your bedroom as well, not to mention a beautiful sight to wake up to.

- Do you find dark and cozy environments more relaxing or open, bright, and airy ones? Which describes your bedroom?

- If daylight streams in through your windows or a skylight and that wakes you, getting new window treatments or moving your bed could help. (I once traced a bout of insomnia to the *blinds* in my bedroom. A new street lamp glared at me from between the slats. I moved the bed and voilà! Sleeplessness *conquered*.)

- Not getting *enough* natural light during your waking hours can make it difficult to shut off at night. Our circadian rhythms are governed by light, and, for some of us, so is our likelihood of sleep-disrupting sadness. Nature gives us light, air, water, and earth every day. It's our job to take these in and use what we need, like bears and other living things, and give back what we can. There are special "natural" lights on the market now that may help you if daylight is scarce in your day.

- Let your mind's eye take over and soothe you with restful images. The vision of a duck's graceful trail through a lake can accompany you to bed. Lull yourself to sleep with sunsets, lazy marshlands, and gently swaying palm trees. (P.S. This is also a good way to destress during the day.)

3. Touch. Are your sheets cool and soft? Cozy but not too hot? Is your bed too firm? Not firm enough? Anything from muscle tension to dry skin could warrant a change in bedding material. A stiff neck could mean your pillow is too fluffy, straining your neck all night long. Some people sleep best with no pillow at all. Pay attention to how your body feels before you get in bed and when you wake up in the morning.

- What kind of clothes do you love to wear during the day? Do you feel perfectly comfortable in the clothes, shoes, undergarments, and socks that you have on right now? The habit of wearing pretty clothes that are uncomfortable during the day can carry into your choice of sleepwear, leaving you less than comfortable in bed. At night, comfort is king.

- Taking a hot shower an hour or two before bedtime raises your body temperature so you'll be slightly chilly by the time you're ready to turn in. This makes crawling under the covers deliciously appealing!!

- Changing sleep positions can affect your sleep. Sleeping on your stomach or curling up into a fetal position can signal your subconscious with a message of sleepiness.

TRUST IN A TEDDY BEAR

You're never too old for a teddy bear or a special pillow.
In today's computerized everything age,
we are all starved for *touch*.

4. Sound. Some people can't sleep a wink when they hear the sound of a TV, while others can't drop off without it. What you hear, or do not hear, can also disturb your sleep.

- Ever notice how the sound of rain bouncing on the leaves of trees can lull you to sleep? Do you sleep better with storms raging outside? How about the sound of waves crashing onto the beach, or the gentle lapping rhythm of low tide?

- Do you sleep best alone or with your mate? If your partner snores (or thrashes around in his or her sleep), your sleep could suffer.

- Does your clock tick loud enough to hear? Is it bothering you?

- Barking dogs can certainly keep you awake at night. If notes and kind phone calls to their owners haven't helped, ear plugs or an electric fan might block the noise. (Incidentally, earplugs are great hotel companions too!)

- Sometimes it can be too quiet. If you're used to the presence of subtle sounds, like your dog softly snoring at the foot of your bed, distant traffic sounds, or the occasional bird chirp, pure silence can be distracting.

- Do you find it easier to doze off during a boring movie, or does elevator music lull you to sleep? (Someone once told me the quiet hum of her computer works every time!) Some of us need silence for sleep, and others do not. The next time your eyelids get heavy, note the sounds, or lack thereof, around you.

5. Taste. Let *your taste buds* lure you to sleep?! Read on.

- Mom was right: brush your teeth before bed. Brushing with the same toothpaste or gargling with the same mouthwash each evening can signal your taste buds that it's bedtime.

- A cup of water on your nightstand is a great way to avoid dry mouth...and having to get up for a drink in the early a.m. hours.

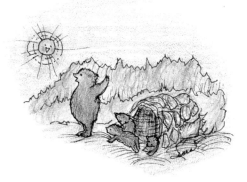

A mother bear digs her den not only as a safe place in which to sleep,
but also as a shelter where she can give birth.

Each of us can do this for ourselves.

Our bedrooms are a safe place where we can
dream about our contributions
to the world and the steps we can take to make them real.

3. Listen to Your Chattering Mind

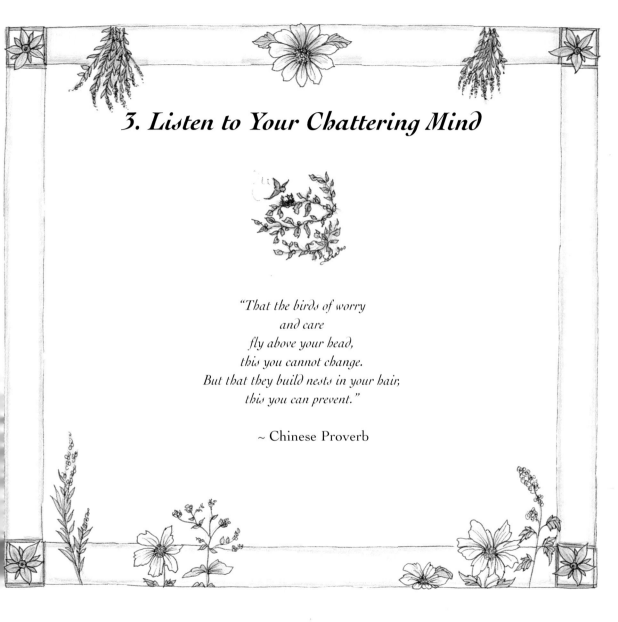

"That the birds of worry
and care
fly above your head,
this you cannot change.
But that they build nests in your hair,
this you can prevent."

~ Chinese Proverb

Insomnia as Teacher

If you're trying to get some sleep and your busy brain won't slow down, there's a reason. It's trying to tell you something.

Let your overactive mind work *for* you. The next night that you cannot sleep, instead of trying to silence your chattering mind, *listen to it*. What are you chattering about?

Much of the spin cycle of anxious thought is caused by conflicting goals:

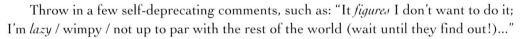

"I *should* do this."
"I *have* to do that."
versus
"But I don't *want* to do either."

Throw in a few self-deprecating comments, such as: "It *figures* I don't want to do it; I'm *lazy* / wimpy / not up to par with the rest of the world (wait until they find out!)..."

blah
blah
blah

And voilà! You have a veritable smorgasbord of nocturnal alarms.

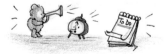

A Tip to Relieve "If I Do 1,000 Things, It Will All Work Out Okay" Syndrome

(Or how to put it all into perspective, so worry can be replaced with more positive mental tasks.)

If worrying about getting it all done (or the ol' "If I plan it to a T, nothing can go wrong") keeps you awake at night, try this:

The next time you catch yourself worrying ~ *day or night* ~ ask yourself this:

What do I *want* to
give to this world?
What do I want to be remembered for?
How much of what I'm stewing about
directly affects that?
Just think.

Look at the imbalances in your life.
Some worry is good, but too much keeps you off center,
not very natural at all.

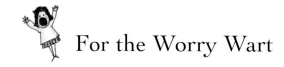

For the Worry Wart

They say 90 percent of what we worry about never comes true, but if you're a worry wart like me, it's that other 10 percent that keeps you anxious!!!!! Especially since you don't necessarily know which 10 percent it will be!

If this sounds like you, take heed. ("Don't *worry!*" doesn't apply here.) There *is* a solution that may work for you.

The Worry Box

Get a pad of paper, a pencil, and a pretty box. (Mine is fabric covered and comfortable looking.) Before bedtime ~ or any time during your busy day ~ make a list of all the things your mind won't let up on: your fears and worries about not getting it all done, about living the life you were meant to (and seemingly are *not*), about the people you love, about work, money, whatever. No fear is too silly or mundane. *Everything* passes "go" here.

Now fold the paper and put it in your box...

Getting into the *habit* of putting your fears to rest in a safe place will help ease your worried mind. The act of writing those fears down *externalizes* them so your *internal peace* has more room to grow *day or night.*

Every once in a while, clean out your box and rid your life of those worries!

(Many thanks to my good friend Betsy for letting me in on this wonderful idea.)

How to Eliminate Anxiety with a To Do List

Preparing a To Do List well before bedtime is a good way to reduce worry.

Time management experts recommend picking two or three things on the list that must be done immediately. If you think it's all important or it wouldn't be on the list in the first place, try to pick *extremely* time sensitive material. You may find that much of the other stuff on the list is just that: stuff.

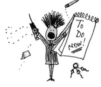

Daily

Go through your To Do List
and check off everything you did today.
Now write down everything
you did that wasn't on the list,
and check them off, too.

Done.

Too often we get so caught up in
worrying about the things
we *didn't* do, we never allow ourselves
the satisfaction of enjoying a sense of accomplishment
about the things we *did* do.

Nurture the habit of looking at today's accomplishments
to foster trust in your abilities for tomorrow.

Mind Balance

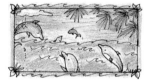

*"I discovered the secret of
the sea in meditation upon
a dewdrop."*

~ Kahlil Gibran

Do you, like so many others, use coffee to help your overwhelmed mind focus and concentrate?

If you're drinking lots of coffee throughout the day up until, say, 2 p.m., you may actually be experiencing a rebound effect of the coffee buzz when you should be sleeping. (Teas, colas, and hot cocoa count too, unless they are marked caffeine free.) If coffee keeps your mental act ultra-focused by day, then it is nighttime when your mind is running free.

Why do you feel you *have to* keep your mind in restraints all day?

Possible reason: You are trying to juggle so many details during an average day that you use caffeine to help you keep them in logical order.

So...How can you stop forcing yourself into artificial highs and lows, and follow your natural rhythms instead?

The Two Sides of Your Mind

THE LEFT SIDE	THE RIGHT SIDE
Concrete	Creative
Logical	Intuitive
Goal oriented	Process oriented
"To Do"	"Could Do"
Black and white	Multihued
Has parameters, rules	Open-ended, goes by gut feelings

Our minds are dual in nature. When one side is suppressed, the other side may kick into overdrive and fill in the gap.

If falling asleep is no problem but staying that way is, your right brain might be trying to push forward some messages or ideas, but, just as they make it to the forefront, your ever-logical left brain kicks in and hushes them up.

Have you ever woken up remembering a strong feeling from a dream, but, try as hard as you might, you just couldn't recall *what happened?*

Dreaming is the right brain's poetry, composed in a sort of hieroglyphics. Dreams are often open-ended and far from logical, their meanings lost on us ~ unless we put some serious effort into deciphering them. When we do attempt to understand their messages, quite often we find solutions to nagging problems that logic alone couldn't solve.

Worrying can become a hobby with insomniacs. Even if you're not consciously obsessing over something as you lie awake, the habitual quest to figure things out before the day is over can send your left brain into fight or flight mode ~ that mental fencing match known as a chattering mind.

It could be that
those running thoughts that *refuse* to
let you sleep are really a creative pursuit
trying to break free.

It's as if the logical side of your brain
won't *shut up,*
and as a result the fuzzy-lined illogical
highly creative side
can't get through.
Hmmm.

What have you dreamed of doing in your lifetime?

If you're sleepwalking through your days,
just going through the motions, you may not
be able to sleep well at night.

Live your days well!

Insomnia can also happen when your creative mind
is telling you something and your logical mind
is trying to figure it out,
which is kind of like
trying to dissect an orange
with an apple
core.

(?!?)
Pretty
hard
to
do.

How do you bring more balance to your mind? The solution is twofold:

1. Exercise that stiff old right brain during waking hours so your poor left brain can take a long-needed rest at night (and stop chattering for a while).

2. Offer your left brain some form of daily release.

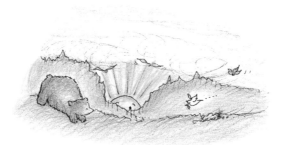

A very good friend of mine has fallen asleep for years while entertaining the very thoughts many insomnia experts say will keep us awake: attempts to resolve a perplexing work problem.

My friend claims he wakes with a solution every time he does this. Why? Because he *trusts* that he will have a *solution* when he wakes up.

Without that *trust*
this thought process is
wildly distracting
~ from sleep, from rest, from peace of mind.

With this trust, however, sleep becomes an unconscious opportunity to allow your logical side to rest and let your creative subconscious work on a big problem, or a lot of little ones.

The answers may come in small pieces — LITTLE ANSWERS to BIG PROBLEMS that add up to *the answer*. It takes time and patience to exercise your mind this way, but it will get easier and let you rest peacefully.

When Your Mind Just Won't Stop Chattering

*B*e patient with yourself, even if you're only *pretending*.

This is tough stuff. You probably have given up on good sleep, losing patience with yourself long ago. That's understandable.

Acknowledge your impatience with your sleeping patterns (or rather, lack thereof). When you can't sleep *again,* get up and pretend you're feeding a hungry baby:

there's nothing you can do right at this moment to prevent it;
accept it
and feed the kid.

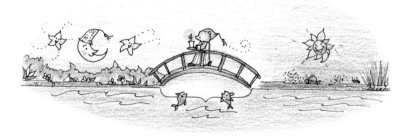

Respect your chattering mind. This is a part of you, trying to be heard.

Listen.

> *"Wretched and barren is the*
> *discontent that quarrels*
> *with its tools instead of*
> *with its skill."*
>
> ~ J. Martineau

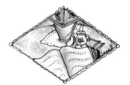

Your body wants to sleep. But your mind won't let you. Leave your bedroom and occupy your mind in a manner that *empties* it:

- Zone out with a relaxing (or boring) book. It's not a bad idea to have a book just for bedtime reading. This way you subtly remind yourself it is time to go to sleep. News and glitzy magazines may keep your mind churning; if you find them too stimulating, save them for daytime when you're *trying* to stay awake.

- Let your eyes do your unwinding for you! Browse through the beautiful pictures in those calendars and coffee table books you rarely take the time to look at.

- A great way to get in touch with yourself is by keeping a personal journal. Writing about the nitty-gritty of how you *really* feel about what happened at work today, or back when your parents divorced, or when your pet died is soul-lightening stuff. Getting into the habit of putting your feelings on paper can be a rewarding, healthy part of your day.

Again, the goal is to empty your overflowing mind.

This new practice may take several nights to work.
The important thing to remember,
though, is to choose mental activities that have a *releasing effect,*
and not to fill your chattering mind
with more stuff to chatter about.

Plan for your insomnia.
Make a comfortable place for yourself.

Have a book ready,
your journal handy,
some art or sewing supplies out.

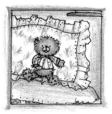

A Few Last Resorts

Think of the things that have made you nod off in the past *involuntarily.*

- Boring meetings? Long-winded teachers?
    - ~You can now purchase videos of some of the most boring college lectures around!

- Study hall? The library?
    - ~ Buy a used textbook today!

- Someone's family videos? (Certainly not your own!)
    - ~ Ask for a copy today. They'll be *thrilled!* (Just don't tell them *why.)*

- Air travel?
    - ~ Can't help you there.

Fill in the blank:

_____

_____

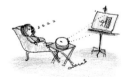

If all else fails, whip out the ol' slide projector and let 'er rip !!!

Animal behavior can yield tremendous tips about how to live by our internal nature and not in friction against it.

If you have a pet
watch him sleep.

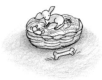

A cat's slowly blinking eyes or the gentle rise and fall of a dog's belly will plant a soothing picture in your psyche.

Watch how your pets operate during the day, too.
Animals don't push themselves unless it's for something they really want
~ whether it's a Frisbee, a treat, or a pat on the head.

Deep Beneath the Surface

*"As he thinketh in his heart,
so is he."*

~ Proverbs 23:7

In nature we find evidence of forces out of control due to imbalances far beneath the earth's surface.

Tsunami literally means "harbor wave" in Japanese and is the scourge of coastlines throughout the Pacific. Caused by a disturbance beneath the ocean floor ~ such as an earthquake ~ a tsunami is a long and lateral force. Most tsunami are barely three feet high far out on the ocean. But the wave rises as it nears the shallow-floored coastline and bucks up from the sheer force of impact, unfolding like an accordion onto the land.

Chronic insomnia can be caused by an issue buried deep in your psyche that, until now, you have been unable to deal with: a death, a childhood trauma, a failed relationship, or illness.

All of nature's creatures have defenses to protect them from harm, and we are no exception. Shielding your conscious mind from the unthinkable is both reasonable and necessary, for a while.

But sooner or later the tsunami hits shore.

If you suspect that such an event is contributing to your sleeplessness, a skilled therapist can help you through it. A support group for your specific trauma can also be highly beneficial. The only way to end an emotional tsunami is to deal with it on the surface, consciously "weather it," so to speak.

All the world feels better after a storm has passed, and you will too.

It may seem like I am saying,
"Fix your whole life and learn to love
yourself unconditionally, and then
you will be able to sleep."
But I'm not.

I am saying that, even though your insomnia may seem uncontrollable, focusing on the things you *can* do ~ small, positive, self-affirming habits ~ will increase your sense of internal power, and that will bring you

a very
personal
peace.

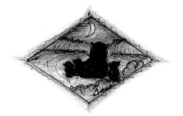

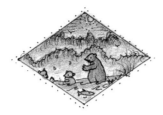

Bears don't worry about looking foolish while they slap and splash to find fish; their style is all their own. But at the same time fishing is serious business to a bear.

Catch or starve.

In nature daily life is neither judged nor measured, and the outcome always ~ in one form or another ~ nourishes the planet's balance.

Imagine not *having* to be good at what you are doing. Picture just doing something for the joy of it, the *unjudged* challenge of it, to satisfy the curiosity it piques in you.

If you concentrate on what you are doing and how you feel while you are doing it, moment by moment adjustments can be made. Solutions, then, become an integral part of how you live your life.

This is "Creative Problem Solving Nature's Way." As you develop this habit of approaching problems, obstacles, and imbalances in your life in small, incremental doses, you may find that the bulk of your energy is being used constructively, while destructive habits like self-criticism and worrying yourself awake get crowded out.

In other words, if you expend all your energy living a life based upon *your* values ~ *authentically your own* ~ your mind and body will be spent and ready to rest at night.

Nature Can't Be Timed

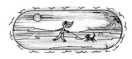

he next time
you go for a walk
or work out
or do anything physical,
don't time yourself
or count repetitions.
Walk quickly or slowly,
whatever is most comfortable for you.
What emotions are you feeling?
Check in with your body occasionally.
Is your breathing labored or steady?
How do your legs,
arms, shoulders, and neck feel?
Adjust your pace accordingly.
Become aware of what this movement
is doing for your mind and body,
and stop when you have had enough.

You have just practiced living in accordance to your natural rhythms
~ in mind *and* body.

BEAR FACT

Since ancient times, the bear has symbolized rebirth, emerging from darkness into a whole new world.

- Once you begin to delve beneath the surface of your chattering mind, which has been keeping you awake, you will find aspects of yourself that will surprise you, delight you, and perhaps even frighten you.

- One thing is certain: your insomnia is here to teach you something about *you* ~ the real you. You may already know what is out of balance in your life; now is the time to begin digging through it and incorporate what you find into your new approach to life.

You are on the verge of something great: a re-creation of *you*.

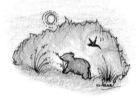

INSOMNIA FOOTNOTE

How can pursuing a passion heal your insomnia?
Our passions heal us by requiring us to overcome whatever
is holding us back from living a satisfying life. Imagine the ways
your passions can bring a wholeness to your waking life, so that
sleeping well can become the norm in your nighttime hours.

Make Your Chattering Mind Work for You

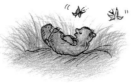

1. Write down your life's goals. This is the Big Stuff:

• The things you'd regret not doing, *not trying to the fullest,* before your time on earth is up.

• The personal characteristics you already have ~ or have a glimmer of ~ that you'd like to develop in your lifetime, i.e., the person you *know* you can become.

2. Each night as you lie in bed (hoping for sleep!), *visualize.*

See yourself in the course of an average day,
doing the big stuff
living a full life
being the best you can be.

You may want to be a farmer, or a great parent, or a pastry chef, or a builder of magnificent homes. Your goal can be anything beneficial to you and to your world. (*Hint:* Your world, our world, *always* benefits from your talents and good will.)

Now see yourself at the end of such a fulfilling day, crawling into bed and falling fast asleep, waking rested and refreshed the following morning.

If you do what's *really* important to you
today,
everything you need for tomorrow
will be available to you.

Take a *tiny* step:

- Read a book on how to write the screenplay that's gnawing at you. (Michael Hauge's *Writing Screenplays That Sell* is excellent!)

- Talk to an entrepreneur about the business you dream of starting.

- Call the chamber of commerce in the place you'd *really* love to live.

This is imperative. However small an action you take, you must do it to prove to yourself that you are serious about your pursuits, that you are trustworthy with *your* stuff. (You are with everyone else's!)

Bears don't pass up the perfect spot for their den out of some sense of obligation to the other bears. They take it and build the best den they can, with the materials they have available.

Flowers never apologize for growing, nor should you.
Nature never wants *that*.

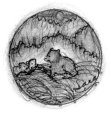

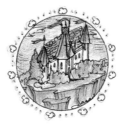

"If you have built castles in the air,
your work need not be lost; that is where
they should be. Now put foundations under them."

~ Henry David Thoreau

The Hopi believe the Creator bestows upon each of us a special gift or talent, or perhaps several smaller ones, and through the practice of this gift we give our unique form of love to the universe.

In effect, practicing our craft is synonymous with allowing a Higher Power to work *through* us. To avoid searching for and using one's special gifts is to reject divine intent, and love, and life at its best. Unearthing our talents brings meaning and balance to our lives.

"Teachers open the door,
but you must enter by yourself."

~ Chinese Proverb

Food for the Right Side of Your Brain

Your left brain has served you well all these years. So well, in fact, that it may have taken over.

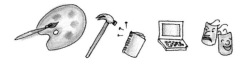

If you do nothing else after reading this book
but pursue a personal goal
~ whether it be an old interest or a new one ~
you have succeeded.
Any time you do something that requires you to take a chance

and let go of a cut-and-dry result,
you are reestablishing your trust in yourself.

You may have an image in your mind's eye
of what a finished painting "should" look like,
and you may even be able to reproduce that vision on canvas.

Give up these expectations.
Let your moment-by-moment decision making determine
what colors you use, what brush or sponge you pick up.

You will experience delight in unexpected ways.
By just letting go you'll be learning
to allow that deep, all-natural part of you to run free.

Your personal truth is what matters.
When you live according to that truth you will achieve sleepy-time peace.

4. Weather the Storm

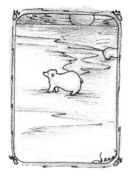

How does a polar bear deal with a storm?
He literally turns his back to it.

torms in polar bear country can be brutal, as you can probably imagine. But in the face of an arctic blast of ice and snow, a polar bear will lie down in the direction opposite to the strongest wind and wait until it has passed. When it's over, he will dig himself out and move on in search of food.

But when the sun is out, you might catch a polar bear lying there, paws splayed and legs outstretched, soaking up the sunshine.

When the world is just too much, wait out the storm. Sometimes the only option is to save up your strength for the good days. Eventually the storm will pass.

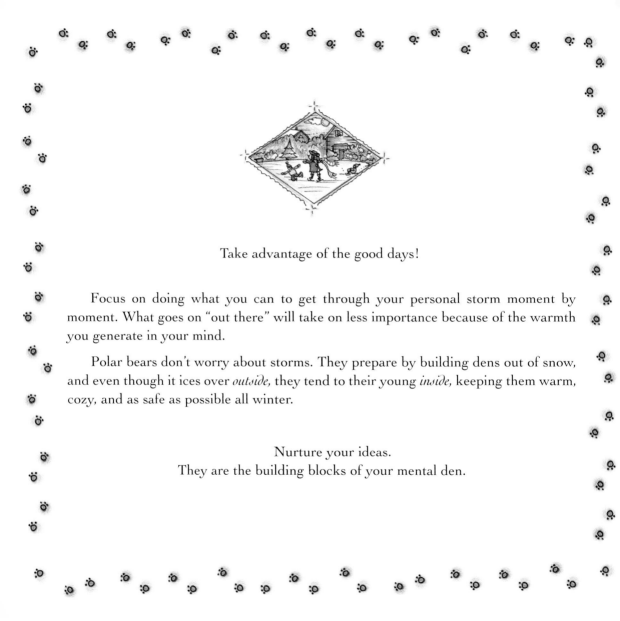

Take advantage of the good days!

Focus on doing what you can to get through your personal storm moment by moment. What goes on "out there" will take on less importance because of the warmth you generate in your mind.

Polar bears don't worry about storms. They prepare by building dens out of snow, and even though it ices over *outside,* they tend to their young *inside,* keeping them warm, cozy, and as safe as possible all winter.

Nurture your ideas.
They are the building blocks of your mental den.

There Are Two Plans of Attack

PLAN A

1. Get the "stuff" of your day out ~ on paper, in the gym, or in a therapist's office or other safe place. (Not on the road, please!)

2. Unwind with a hot bath or a good book (self-help, inspirational, fiction ~ something *positive*). Pray or meditate before you go to sleep.

    Spend a few minutes doing whatever brings you peace.

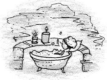

3. Most important ~

If you can't sleep, *don't try.*
Do what you can. Make *rest* your goal instead.

Did you ever see a dog lying, eyes wide, chin on paw, pondering?
He's just resting. That's okay, too...*just drifting.*

But what if you find "just drifting" to be a maddening concept (or just not possible)?
If you're thinking, "If I could just drift off, I wouldn't have a sleep problem,
right?" then you might try...

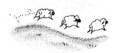

PLAN B

Reverse the strategy (sort of).

In *Do One Thing Different,* author Bill O'Hanlon tells us about one of his psycho-therapy instructors, Milton Erickson, who had a patient with hopeless insomnia. Ever since his wife had died years earlier, the man couldn't sleep. Erickson told the man to lie in bed and, if he still couldn't sleep in fifteen minutes, to get up and do something he *hated* to do: clean his hardwood floors.

By the third night the man fell asleep right away. The connection his subconscious made with insomnia and something he hated to do was critical.

Think of something *you* hate to do.

The next time you cannot sleep, get up and do it. Keep working at it until morning. Make insomnia *so unpleasant* for yourself that the inner you will take over and say,

"Hey, I'm ready for bed."

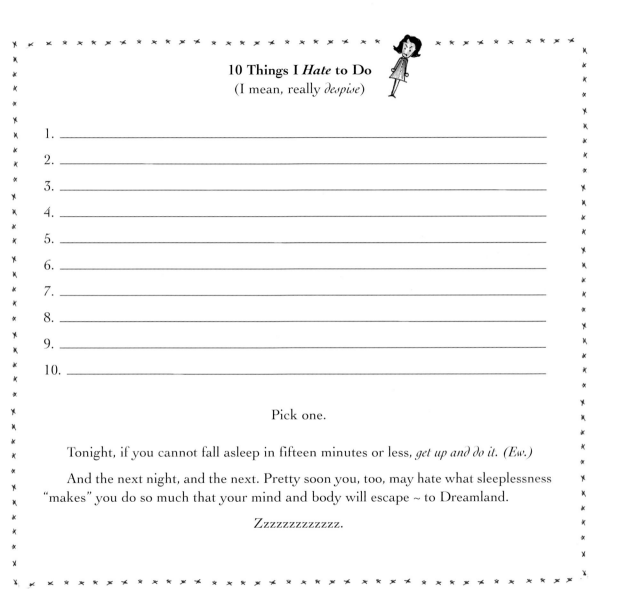

10 Things I *Hate* to Do
(I mean, really *despise*)

1. _____
2. _____
3. _____
4. _____
5. _____
6. _____
7. _____
8. _____
9. _____
10. _____

Pick one.

Tonight, if you cannot fall asleep in fifteen minutes or less, *get up and do it. (Ew.)*

And the next night, and the next. Pretty soon you, too, may hate what sleeplessness "makes" you do so much that your mind and body will escape ~ to Dreamland.

Zzzzzzzzzzzz.

HINT: A GOOD WAY TO TELL WHICH PLAN (A OR B) IS GOOD FOR YOU

Think of something you attempted to do recently that you just couldn't do. Frustrating, huh? Okay, now think: How did you overcome your difficulty ~ leave it for later, punch a pillow and force yourself to go back to it, or fiddle with it fruitlessly? If you're a pillow puncher or a fruitless fiddler, Plan B may be for you. If you left it for later, Plan A may be your best bet. Try 'em both and see.

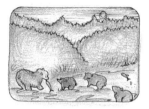

BEAR FACT

Grizzlies have different fishing styles, each one unique. Some stand at the river bank and catch fish with their sharp-clawed paws, while others jump right in and catch fish in the water.

INSOMNIA FOOTNOTE

Find your sleep style. Start by noticing what soothes you and helps you unwind during the day. What you discover may be an essential component of what helps you relax at night. Your insomnia is with you for a reason, and you can only benefit from getting to know yourself better.

If You Can't Sleep at Night, Take a Closer Look at Your Evenings

1. Look at what you are currently doing.

What did you do last night during the hours prior to bedtime? Note any catnaps on a train or bus on the commute home from work, or the flurry of activity you were caught up in late at night, either of which can delay your internal cues to go to sleep.

2. Think of what you can do differently.

Think of what you can add to your life to help release stress from your mind and body. Destressing by day can definitely add peace to your nights. It's much more relaxing to think of the pleasant things you can do rather than those things you must give up. Perhaps a good book or lively music can keep you awake on the train so a nap won't disrupt your sleep later on.

Where you sleep can greatly affect *how* you sleep. Some people find it easier to sleep all night on the couch. However, you may be able to doze off in front of the living room TV, but find that waking up and moving to the bedroom is a huge interruption. Establishing a nightly routine will help ease you directly into bed, eliminating the break in your sleep time.

Note to night workers: The suggestions in this book are meant to help you as well! A regular bedtime routine, regardless of what the clock says, is important. Winding down from your workday, sleeping in a comforting space, and avoiding not-so-obvious sleep irritants are vital, no matter what time your lights go out.

BEAR FACT

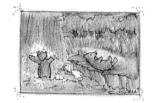

Bears do what bears were meant to do.
Nature gives us all the equipment we need to do what we need to do, including *sleep*.

Physical bodies need to move, barring illness, every day. If you have a desk job or a mostly sedentary lifestyle, you need to make a point of exercising. Insomnia slips away for many insomniacs who take up a regular habit of walking, playing tennis, swimming, biking, or running.

It sounds too simple.
If you want to move less at night,
move more during the day.

"But," you might say, "my body isn't tired. It's my *mind* that won't shut off."

True. But our bodies and our minds are all part of the same package. Think of insomnia as the result of a glitch in one of the two. If our minds won't turn off, *our bodies can help repair the glitch and shut them up.*

If you don't have much time to exercise, try breaking it up throughout the day: ten minutes of calisthenics in the morning and again after work, and a ten- or fifteen-minute walk at lunchtime. (Grabbing a friend to walk along with you can make for good "venting" time, not to mention a laugh or stimulating conversation.)

My Sleep Diary

Keep a sleep diary for at least two weeks to determine what your sleep habits really are. The *practice* of recording your daytime and evening routines can be a great way to track down your sleep demons. What you are creating is *the habit of awareness.*

Wake Up:
I woke up at: _____ *(time).*

I felt: _____ *rested* _____ *cranky* _____ *tired* _____ *sad* _____ *excited* _____ *(fill in)*

My Day:
List what you actually did today, not necessarily what you were "supposed" to do. You can do it hour-by-hour or in list form, whichever is easier for you. What I actually did today:

_____

_____

_____

_____

_____

_____

_____

(Incidentally, if you need several pages to do this part, you may be doing too much.)

My Evening:
This period is from dinnertime until bedtime. List what you ate and drank during and after dinner:

_____

_____

List what you did after dinner, including any work, chores, phone calls, errands, activities, and exercise:

_____

_____

My Bedtime Routine:
Record how and when you prepare for bed. Include baths, showers, activities, and the general mood of your household for an hour or two leading up to bedtime:

_____

_____

Bedtime:
Record how you felt at bedtime, where you went to sleep, how you felt during the night, and what time(s) you woke up and why. If any thoughts kept you awake, record those too:

_____

_____

Wake Up:
Back to the beginning.

Pavlov's Bears

(Okay, so they were dogs.)

P avlov was a famous pioneer in the field of behavioral psychology. He found that ringing a bell before feeding his dogs made them expect dinner every time they heard the bell. The poor pooches would salivate upon hearing the bell, whether food was brought to them or not.

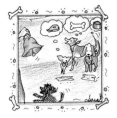

That Pavlov.

Human beings love habit too, so establishing a routine can be very helpful for promoting sleep.

The mere existence of a nightly routine can be
more important than the components of the routine.

Remember to keep as many of the sensory conditions *consistent* as possible each night. Even wearing new pajamas or using a different brand of mouthwash may subconsciously disrupt your sleep.

Focus on these conditions (which you can control) rather than on the one thing you can't seem to do: sleep. Create your own sensory cues to signal your eyes to shut.

Suggestions for a
Pretty Good Nighttime Routine

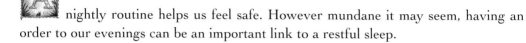
nightly routine helps us feel safe. However mundane it may seem, having an order to our evenings can be an important link to a restful sleep.

ABOUT TWO HOURS BEFORE BED YOU MIGHT...

- Get the day-to-day stuff done (as much as is humanly possible), such as:
    - ~ Bathe the kids and put them to bed
    - ~ Walk the pets
    - ~ Clean up the kitchen

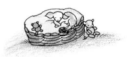

- Relax, unwind, and get comfortable:
    - ~ Take a hot shower
    - ~ Change into comfy sweats (your "wind down" clothes)

- Empty your mind
    - ~ Get your To Do list in order for tomorrow
    - ~ Write in your journal
    - ~ Make a few "deposits" into your Worry Box

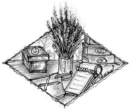

- Engage in nontaxing activities:
    - ~ A small snack
    - ~ Light reading
    - ~ Light TV

- Get ready to sleep:
    - ~ Put on your pajamas
    - ~ Set your alarm
    - ~ Keep a fresh glass of water on your nightstand in case you get thirsty during the night
    - ~ Read a book until you start to nod off

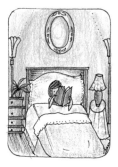

By balancing the components of your current nighttime routine with a few new ones, you now have the tools to create your own version of a good night.

And while you and your partner or family may need time to adjust to your new routine, consider this:

How patient and loving and understanding can you be
when you are chronically sleep deprived?
Now it's time to create a nightly routine that's wonderful for *you.*

Weather the Storm Your Way

What is your idea of a nighttime routine that leads up to a sound night's sleep? It's important to start your reworked evening routine *with where you are now*.

Think of what your evenings are like now on a typical weeknight. Look at your sleep diary for patterns you may be needlessly locked into, and imagine how you could alter your current routine (or lack thereof) to your benefit.

My current routine is:

_____

_____

_____

Three things I *won't* change about my current routine are:

1. _____

2. _____

3. _____

Three things I *could* do to make my nights more sleep conducive are:

1. _____

2. _____

3. _____

5. Mother Yourself to Sleep

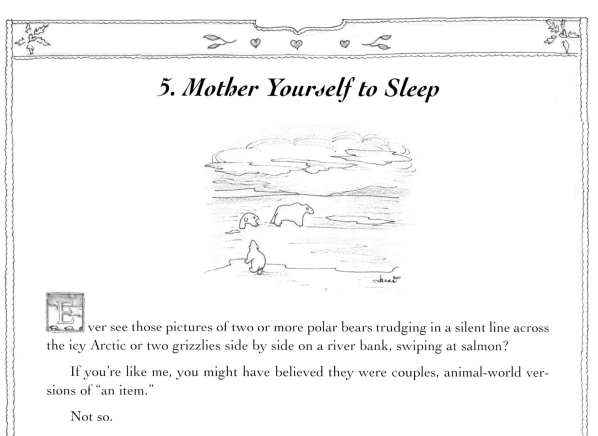

Ever see those pictures of two or more polar bears trudging in a silent line across the icy Arctic or two grizzlies side by side on a river bank, swiping at salmon?

If you're like me, you might have believed they were couples, animal-world versions of "an item."

Not so.

Those are pictures of a mother and child.

Mother polar bears care for their young for at least the first two years of life. Grizzly mothers also remain quite close to their cubs, teaching them by imitation how to catch salmon and forage for nuts, berries, and delicious plants. It must be quite a task for Mama Grizzly to watch her frisky cubs while trying to catch fish with her bare paws.

A Mother's Love

Is the kind of love we all need.

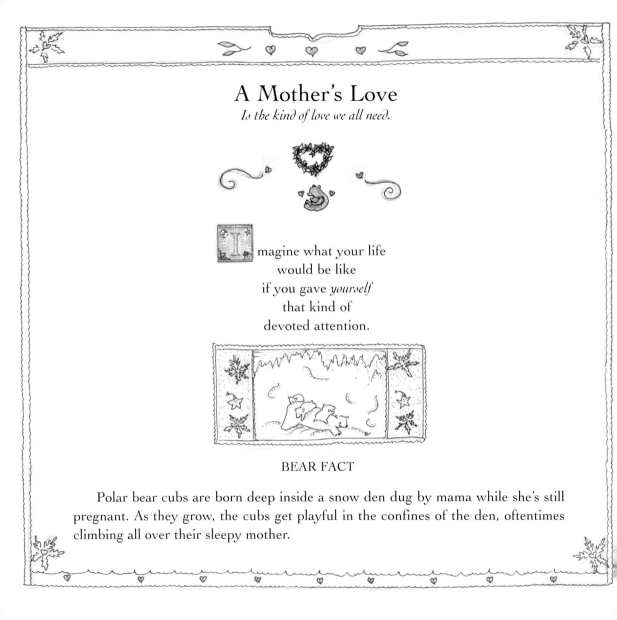

Imagine what your life
would be like
if you gave *yourself*
that kind of
devoted attention.

BEAR FACT

Polar bear cubs are born deep inside a snow den dug by mama while she's still pregnant. As they grow, the cubs get playful in the confines of the den, oftentimes climbing all over their sleepy mother.

10 Ways I Could Play More in My Life Today

"But still you will sometimes find the Raven and Grizzly Bear together, making medicine to help others, or sometimes just fooling around together in Nature, trying to outdance each other along the river or creek."

~ Bobby Lake-Thom,
Spirits of the Earth

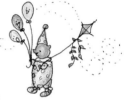

All animals play. Humans must, too.

1. _____

2. _____

3. _____

4. _____

5. _____

6. _____

7. _____

8. _____

9. _____

10. _____

Pamper Your Dampened Spirit

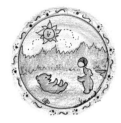

When was the last time
you laughed from deep down
in your belly, the kind of laugh
that makes your sides ache and
your eyes tear and that tickles your
very spirit?

Vow to watch a funny movie or TV show or
read a very funny book.

Or best of all,
spend time with a really funny friend.

BEAR FACT

When a bear is angry, you know it.

Occasionally a grizzly will charge ~ sometimes bluffing, sometimes not. But when cornered or threatened, a bear will stand up on his haunches and roar, mouth open, snout raised, ears flattened back against his head, or he may simply shake his head back and forth and keep his roar to himself. Either way, there's no missing when a bear is angry.

With us humans, however, it's a different story. From the time we were very young children some of us were taught (directly or indirectly) that showing our emotions ~ especially anger ~ is wrong, or ugly, or unacceptable. Of course we can't go through life roaring at people or charging at annoying coworkers (although, *can you imagine?!*), but stuffed anger is bound to come out ~ sometimes in the form of worry, or anxiety, or passive hostility, or even in the form of being too "good" all the time (and suffering the consequences later).

Let yourself *feel* your emotions.

Rather than lashing outward (being mean to others) or lashing inward (being mean to yourself), sit with your anger and feel it burn and tingle at every pore. You may not be able to do this for very long.

Then let yourself cry: big, bawling sobs. Beneath most anger are fear and grief, but we tend to lash out ~ or in ~ to get rid of it. Be with your emotions. Yell in the car about what *really* makes you mad. (Hint: It may have nothing to do with traffic.) Cry your eyes out in a big, fluffy pillow. Let out the difficult feelings but practice sharing the fun feelings, too. *Express* your enthusiasm about something with a like-minded person.

A rock in a flowing river is never an obstacle; the water runs *around it.*

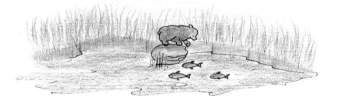

Learning to be nice to yourself is a skill that can carry you past the tough parts of life, including your current struggles with insomnia. It's something we insomniacs (and sleepers, too) need to do anyway, so why not learn to love yourself and care about yourself?

That's something you *can* do, starting right now.

A Lesson in Love and Self-Kindness

"How do I love thee?
Let me count the ways."

~ Elizabeth Barrett Browning

I don't know how you love yourself. This is very individual, something you come to on your own. But I do know a good way to start the process: Practicing *self-kindness*.

- Tell yourself it's okay when you begin to feel panic or dread when you make a mistake. (We all do!)

- Set up a private place to unwind in, or to sit quietly in, for ten minutes every day.

- Listen to your inner voice ~ your gut ~ and act on what it says. Listen and follow.

- Focus on the *good* things, the things you like about yourself. You deserve your respect!

So, how do you love yourself? You come up with the ways.

"You will find it less easy to uproot faults, than to choke them by gaining virtues. Do not think of your faults; still less of others' faults; in every person who comes near you look for what is good and strong: honor that; rejoice in it; and, as you can, try to imitate it; and your faults will drop off, like dead leaves, when their time comes."

~ J. Ruskin

Make a list of ten things you could do
to treat yourself *better.*

It could be something big, like "Take the breaks I need during the workday," or something small, like "Pick a flower or buy one for the dinner table tonight."

1. _____

2. _____

3. _____

4. _____

5. _____

6. _____

7. _____

8. _____

9. _____

10. _____

Now pick one thing and do it or part of it, *today*. (If you "forget" ~ ha! ~ just think about doing it. Picture yourself doing it, and relaxing happily.)

A mother panda bear usually has only one cub, born about the size of a hamster. She holds her baby in her arms *constantly* until he is a few weeks old. Like other bears, the panda is a truly devoted mother, nursing and protecting her cub, and later showing him how to feed and fend for himself until he is ready to go off on his own, when he is about a year and a half old.

Be a mother bear to yourself!

Your Plan of Action Thus Far Is...

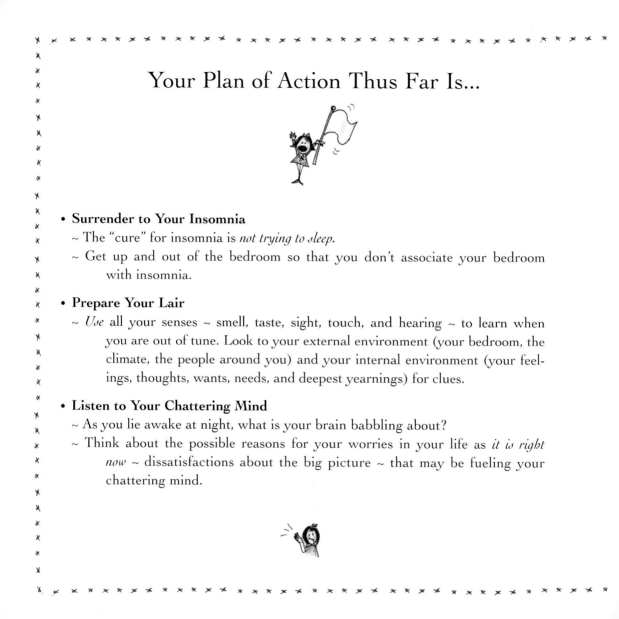

- **Surrender to Your Insomnia**
  - ~ The "cure" for insomnia is *not trying to sleep*.
  - ~ Get up and out of the bedroom so that you don't associate your bedroom with insomnia.

- **Prepare Your Lair**
  - ~ *Use* all your senses ~ smell, taste, sight, touch, and hearing ~ to learn when you are out of tune. Look to your external environment (your bedroom, the climate, the people around you) and your internal environment (your feelings, thoughts, wants, needs, and deepest yearnings) for clues.

- **Listen to Your Chattering Mind**
  - ~ As you lie awake at night, what is your brain babbling about?
  - ~ Think about the possible reasons for your worries in your life as *it is right now* ~ dissatisfactions about the big picture ~ that may be fueling your chattering mind.

- **Honor Your Insomnia**
  - ~ *Plan for sleepless nights.*
  - ~ Think of your insomnia as a teacher, trying to tell you that something needs your attention.
  - ~ *Practice* trusting the natural flow of things. Do everyday things in a different order, in whatever order you feel like doing them, instead of in the order you think you must do them.
  - ~ Watch how children play. They make the most of what is around them at any given moment by receiving what life deals out and working with that, instead of trying to predict the outcome. This may seem like an illogical way of doing some things, but it is the greenhouse in which trust, satisfaction, and self-generated peace can grow.

- **Weather the Storm**
  - ~ *Get your stress out.*
  - ~ Physically: through exercise and more general *movement during the day*. You *must* have an escape route for all the anger, frustration, and nervous energy that life can generate.
  - ~ Mentally: on paper, in your journal, on a splashy, splotchy canvas, in words or in pictures, and into your Worry Box (if it will fit!).
  - ~ *Have a nighttime routine.* Ready your body and mind for bed *your way.*

- **Mother Yourself to Sleep**
  - ~ Be gentle with yourself ~ mentally, physically, and spiritually.
  - ~ Let yourself laugh more, feel more, play more.

IV. Remedies

he only rule of thumb I have found from speaking to insomniacs
about what helps them sleep is there *is* no rule of thumb.
(How frustrating is that?!)

What keeps some people hopelessly awake
~ listening to music, surfing the Net, taking hot baths ~
soothes others to a sound sleep.

You need to find what soothes you. Constantly talking or thinking about what you
can't do will keep you stuck. However, talking with others who have *conquered
insomnia* may help you discover an idea that works for you.

And don't just talk to them about their nights. (If they're sleeping,
they can't tell you much.) Find out how they wind down for bed.
And ask them about how they spend their *days:*

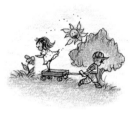

~ Do they exercise?
~ Eat wholesome foods?
~ Eat larger meals at lunch?
~ Read before bed?
~ Ban TV in the bedroom?
~ Love or hate their work?
~ Have more *fun* than you do?

Life is for learning. Let your insomnia be a bridge to what others can teach you.

Practice Relaxing During the Day

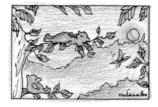

"Merciful powers, restrain me in the cursed thoughts that nature gives way to in repose!"

~ William Shakespeare,
Macbeth

or five minutes, sit comfortably
and envision the tension in your body
and all the stresses that put it there

evaporating like steam
out of you.

If a chattering mind is a sign of anxiety, and anxiety is primarily worrying about the past (what you *should* have done) and/or agonizing about the future (what you will *have to do*), then quieting your mind involves coming to terms with your *present*.

Let your body help ease your mind.

Yoga and meditation of even the simplest kind can be extremely beneficial to insomniacs. They teach us how to stop the fast-forward and rewind mechanism that fuels our chattering mind, and let us settle down into a state of calm. Learning to breathe correctly while relaxing your muscles is a vital component of the myriad types of yoga you can try.

Believe me, I know how hard this is. The first time I took a meditation and bodywork class it seemed as if the speed of my thoughts *increased* instead of decreased. Against the backdrop of the instructor's soothing voice and the deep breathing of my classmates, my mind raced from one screaming To Do to the next. Even the most stress-free setting in the world couldn't relax me. And, in the absence of external stresses, I had to look at the real source of my anxiety: my worrying, frazzled mind.

That, in itself, was my teacher.

Massage: A Comforting Footnote

"The best way to health is a fragrant bath and an aromatic massage every day."

~ Hippocrates

Massage, by definition, is the manipulation of muscle and tissue to free up blocked energy channels to alleviate whatever ails you ~ from body aches to insomnia. Here are a few of the major types of massage:

1. Swedish massage is probably the most familiar. The massage therapist kneads, drums, and applies pressure to your body to help relax you. Aromatherapy includes massaging essential oils into problematic areas while using these techniques.

2. Deep-tissue and trigger-point massage are used frequently on athletes. These are deeper forms of massage more suitable for loosening up specific muscles.

3. Shiatsu uses concentrated finger pressure, called acupressure. Shiatsu takes deep-tissue massage a bit further, since it treats not only the sore spot, but the entire meridian (energy channel) as well.

4. Bodywork is a type of massage therapy based on the belief that the way we move in daily living can cause or aggravate what ails us. A certified bodywork practitioner will guide you toward healthier, kinder ways to move throughout the day so you function *with* your environment and not in reaction to it.

5. Reflexology and other forms of energy healing are, quite literally, hands-on approaches to healing. The practitioner "feels" where your energy is blocked and places her hands there, sending *Qi* (energy) to open the ailment-causing gap.

Just Add Water

According to traditional Chinese medicine, as learned in the introduction, insomnia is caused by a fire imbalance in the system. Therefore, adding *water* to your lifestyle can help tame this misdirected energy within you.

- Go for a swim, walk near the ocean, or take a warm bath.

- Limit your intake of caffeine and very high protein meals (both of which have a diuretic, or dehydrating, effect).

- Try boiling, braising, poaching, or steaming your food instead of frying, grilling, broiling, or baking it all the time.

- Eat more fruits and veggies, and drink at least a liter of water a day. (A liter sounds like a lot, but it's really only a few glasses ~ about what the average person loses per day just during normal respiration.)

The human body has roughly the same percentage of water as does the earth. It makes sense, then, that if you want more equilibrium in your everyday life, *just add water.*

What's Watsu?

*"I tell my clients just before I pick them up in the water that,
for the next fifty minutes, all they have to do is breathe."*

~ Patricia A. Schmidt, Watsu therapist

Watsu is a gentle form of massage done in a pool of water. I spoke with Patricia Schmidt, a certified Watsu practitioner in Hillsborough, North Carolina, and she explained it this way:

"Imagine being cradled in a practitioner's arms, and the healing magic of your body is surrounded by the gentle flow in a warm-water pool. The client is fully supported, while the practitioner is moving and gently stretching, flexing, and massaging the client's body. The entire process encourages release and relaxation of body, mind, and spirit."

But how can, say, a 4:00 p.m. Watsu appointment help you sleep at midnight? Doing any activity that relaxes both your body and your mind with some consistency will remind your inner resources that this serenity can recur. You may not have felt peaceful in a long time, but the soothing effects of Watsu can awaken that feeling.

If yoga sounds too ambitious and acupuncture scares you, Watsu or other types of massage may be a better choice for you. All you have to do is lie there, aaaahhh!

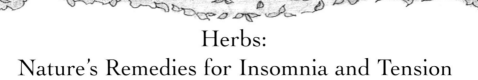

Herbs:
Nature's Remedies for Insomnia and Tension

Many of the herbs on this page can be used to make tea. It is best to have a cup about an hour or two before bed, as part of your nightly routine. Simply steep the herb in boiled water for one to five minutes, and sweeten with a teaspoon of honey or sugar if desired. Some herbs can be purchased in tea bags at your local health food store, or you can grow your own.

Keep in mind that herbs are Mother Nature's drugs. Always check with your doctor before taking any herbal concoction. This is especially important for children, the elderly, and anyone with allergies or compromised immune systems. Bears and other animals may know instinctively what herbs to avoid, but we humans have a ways to go.

Once you get the okay, *always* start with a weak tea or a small dose! Sweet dreams!

Lavender

Passion Flower

Catnip

Evening Primrose

Valerian

Pasque Flower

Heather

Rosemary

Hops

Lemon Balm

Dill

Chamomile

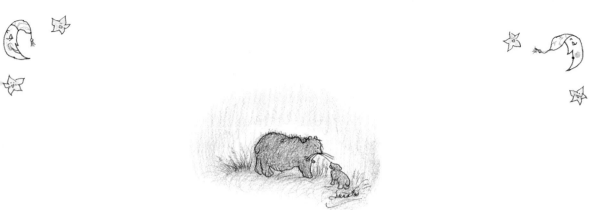

Nature offers her guests some other little helpers:

- For mild insomnia, centuries-old Chinese medicine prescribes a pillow filled with gypsum to relax you with its anxiety-reducing properties.

- Herbalist Ann Jones told me that one of her clients swears massaging lavender-scented oil onto her baby's feet helps him sleep fitlessly through the night. (Grandmother knew what she was doing with all those pretty lavender sachets in her closet…) *Note:* It is crucial to check with your child's doctor before employing herbal oils or remedies.

- According to Ayurvedic medicine, bending forward and brushing your hair earthward calms the spirit and empties the mind for sleep.

Food as Medicine

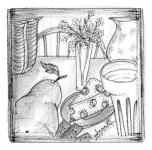

 am a big fan of food as medicine. (Maybe it's because aspirin gives me heartburn, ibuprofen makes me sleepy, store-bought sleeping pills zonk me out for days, and then ~ *zoink!* ~ the rebound effect leaves me drawing sheep on a scratch pad in the living room at 3 a.m.)

Calcium and tryptophan can be a big help. Try designing a snack that contains them as part of your nightly routine. Choose low-fat or nonfat items; heavy foods put the digestive system to work, and fat takes a long time to digest. (Remember, we want *all* parts to relax at night.)

Be sure to eat some fat during the day. Eating a virtually fat-free diet can disrupt sleep also. Fat is a necessary ingredient in the workings of hormones, and we know what it's like when those hormones aren't humming along as they should.

Calcium Can Help You Sleep

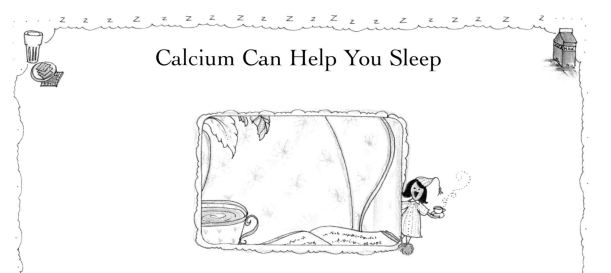

Mothers and grandmothers through the ages have prescribed warm milk as a soothing nightcap for its warming effect on the body, mind, and soul, and for good reason. The *tryptophan* in milk can actually make you drowsy. The *calcium* in milk may add to the equation, along with the vitamin D (the same stuff in sunshine).

Warm milk
can help you sleep.
Try warm milk with a dash of cinnamon or nutmeg.

Some Surprising Sources of Calcium

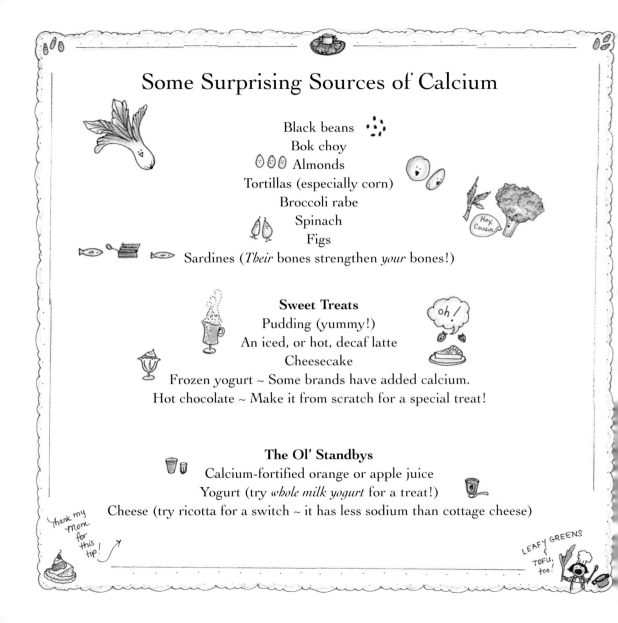

Black beans
Bok choy
Almonds
Tortillas (especially corn)
Broccoli rabe
Spinach
Figs
Sardines (*Their* bones strengthen *your* bones!)

Sweet Treats
Pudding (yummy!)
An iced, or hot, decaf latte
Cheesecake
Frozen yogurt ~ Some brands have added calcium.
Hot chocolate ~ Make it from scratch for a special treat!

The Ol' Standbys
Calcium-fortified orange or apple juice
Yogurt (try *whole milk yogurt* for a treat!)
Cheese (try ricotta for a switch ~ it has less sodium than cottage cheese)

thank my mom for this tip!

Hey, Cousin.

oh!

LEAFY GREENS & TOFU, too!

The Tryptophan Solution

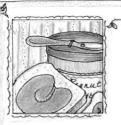
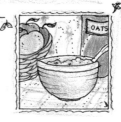

Tryptophan is an amino acid that your body needs in order to make serotonin, the chemical that makes you feel relaxed and happy. If anxiety feeds your insomnia, having a tryptophan-rich snack at least an hour before bedtime can be your food for sleep.

Some Surprising Sources of Tryptophan
(No need to roast a turkey!!!)
Your nightcap snack can be as simple as:

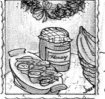
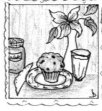

~ Whole grain wheat toast with a thin smear of peanut butter
~ Sliced bananas sprinkled with cinnamon; add a teaspoon
of honey or maple syrup if sugar doesn't bother you at night
~ Cottage cheese on whole grain crackers
~ A warm bowl of oatmeal
~ A raisin bran muffin with a small glass of milk
~ A teacupful of yogurt or skim milk with a graham cracker on the side

Think "whole grain,"
think "dairy,"
think "nut and seed."

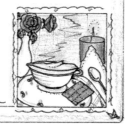

Sweet Tooths Unite!

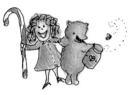

Jean Carper's *Food Pharmacy Guide to Good Eating* claims two spoonfuls of ordinary sugar near bedtime can make you relaxed and drowsy. It's like a drug-free sleeping pill!

Research has shown that sugar and other carbohydrates can increase the level of serotonin ~ the chemical of *calm* ~ in the brain.

A light way to get the sugar (my favorite) is:

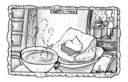

A cup of herbal tea,
with a teaspoon of sugar and warm milk,
and a slice of angel food cake
on the side.

Keep it sugary and light!

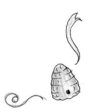

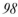

Experiment

Try out different tips and techniques, but always go with your gut. If something isn't working, or if it doesn't agree with you ~ whatever the reason ~ drop it and try something else.

Insomnia is here to tell you something about *yourself*. It's not about what's wrong with you; it's about doing what's *right* for you.

I do hope some of the suggestions in this book have helped you get closer to your own personal solution to more peaceful nights.

May you emerge from the dark winter of insomnia
out into the sweetness of a
well-rested
spring.

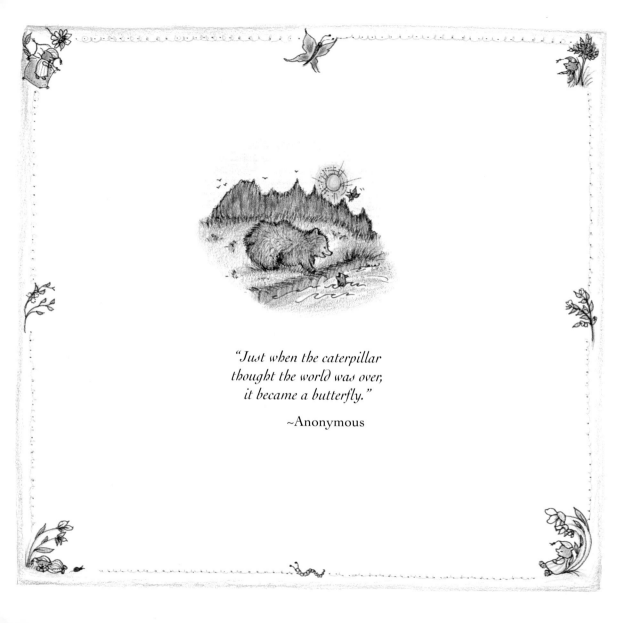

"Just when the caterpillar
thought the world was over,
it became a butterfly."

~Anonymous

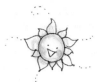

My *New* Sleep Diary

List the three most important things, according to you, that you did today:

_____

_____

_____

List three things you did today to *unwind:*

_____

_____

_____

List three things you do every night as part of your nightly routine:

_____

_____

_____

List three things you'll do with your life once you are sleeping on a regular basis:

_____

_____

_____

Pick one of those things and do it *today.*

_____

V. FURTHER RESOURCES

Sources Used

Carper, Jean. *The Food Pharmacy Guide to Good Eating.* New York: Bantam Books, 1991.

Castleman, Michael. *Nature's Cures.* Emmaus, Pennsylvania: Rodale Press, Inc., 1996.

Estes, Clarissa Pinkola, Ph.D. *Women Who Run with the Wolves.* New York: Ballantine Books, 1992, 1995.

Hauri, Peter, Ph.D., and Shirley Linde, Ph.D. *No More Sleepless Nights.* New York: John Wiley and Sons, Inc., 1990.

Ingall, Marjorie. "How to Get the Sleep of Your Dreams." *New Woman* (December 1999) 96-98.

Lavie, Peretz. *The Enchanted World of Sleep.* New Haven and London: Yale University Press, 1996.

McIntyre, Anne. *The Medicinal Garden.* New York: Henry Holt and Company, Inc., 1997.

McNamara, Sheila. *Traditional Chinese Medicine.* New York: Basic Books, 1996.

O'Hanlon, Bill. *Do One Thing Different.* New York: William Morrow and Co., Inc., 1999.

Pressman, Dr. Alan with Sheila Buff. *The Complete Idiot's Guide to Alternative Medicine.* Indianapolis: Alpha Books, 1999.

Rain, Mary Summer. *Earthway: A North American Visionary's Path to Total Mind, Body, and Spirit Health.* New York: Simon & Schuster, Pocket Books, 1990.

Schmidt, Patricia A. "Watsu Water Therapy Has Many Applications." *Health and Healing in the Triangle,* Chapel Hill, North Carolina: Wellness Communications Inc., (June 2000).

Information for Insomniacs

- **To find a certified acupuncturist near you, contact:**

  National Certification Commission for Acupuncture and Oriental Medicine (NCCAOM)
  11 Canal Plaza, Suite 300
  Alexandria, VA 22314
  (703) 548-9004
  E-mail: info@nccaom.org

- **For more information on insomnia and other sleep disorders, along with other sleep-related information, contact:**

  The National Sleep Foundation
  1522 K Street NW, Suite 500
  Washington, DC 20005
  Fax: (202) 347-3472
  Web site: www.sleepfoundation.org

- **For more information on getting your whole life into a more beautiful balance, read:**

  Alexandra Stoddard's *Gracious Living in a New World* and any of her other books!
  See especially chapter 2, "Reawakening Our Five Senses."

- **For information on Watsu water therapy, call or write:**

  Worldwide Aquatic Bodywork Association
  P.O. Box 889
  Middletown, CA 95461
  (707) 987-3801
  Web site: www.waba.edu

Books on Bears

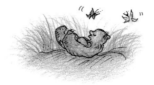

Bailey, Donna, and Christine Butterworth. *Animal World: Bears*. Austin, Texas: Steck-Vaughn Company, 1991.

Bright, Michael. *Project Wildlife: Polar Bear*. New York: Gloucester Press, 1989.

Hillman, James. *Dream Animals*. San Francisco: Chronicle Books, 1997.

Lepthien, Emilie U. *Grizzlies*. New York: Grolier Publishing, Inc., 1996.

Treadwell, Timothy, and Jewel Palovak. *Among Grizzlies: Living with Wild Bears in Alaska*. New York: Harper Collins Publishers, Inc., 1997. (A marvelous book about trust ~ in ourselves, in Nature, and in the merging of the two.)

Xugi, Jin, and Markus Kappeler. *The Giant Panda*. New York: G.P. Putnam's Sons, 1986.

Recommended Reading

Chopra, Deepak, M.D. *Perfect Health*. New York: Harmony Books, 1991.

Hay, Louise L. *You Can Heal Your Life*. Carson, California: Hay House, Inc., 1984, 1987.

Jacobs, Gregg D., Ph.D. *Say Good Night to Insomnia*. New York: Henry Holt and Company, 1998.

Kavasch, E. Barrie, and Karen Baar. *American Indian Healing Arts: Herbs, Rituals and Remedies for Every Season of Life*. New York: Bantam Books, 1999.

Lake-Thom, Bobby. *Spirits of the Earth: A Guide to Native American Nature Symbols, Stories, and Ceremonies*. New York: Plume, 1997.

Maas, Dr. James B. *Power Sleep*. New York: Villard, 1998.

Matthews, A. M. *The Seven Keys to Calm*. New York: Pocket Books, 1997.

Stoddard, Alexandra. *Gracious Living in a New World*. New York: William Morrow and Company, Inc., 1996.